SCOPE AND STANDARDS OF VASCULAR NURSING PRACTICE

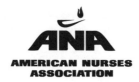

AMERICAN NURSES
ASSOCIATION

nurses
books
.org

The Publishing Program of ANA

Washington, D.C.
2004

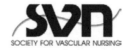

SOCIETY FOR VASCULAR NURSING

Library of Congress Cataloging-in-Publication data

Society for Vascular Nursing (U.S.)
  Scope and standards of vascular nursing practice / Society for Vascular Nursing & American Nurses Association.
    p. ; cm.
Includes bibliographical references and index.
  ISBN 1-55810-221-3
1. Blood-vessels—Diseases—Nursing—Standards.
[DNLM: 1. Vascular Diseases—nursing. 2. Patient Care Planning—standards. WY 152.5 S678s 2004] I. American Nurses Association. II. Title.

RC691.S65 2004
616.1'30231—dc22

                    2004006953

The American Nurses Association (ANA) is a national professional association. This ANA publication—*Scope and Standards of Vascular Nursing Practice*—reflects the thinking of the nursing profession on various issues and should be reviewed in conjunction with state board of nursing policies and practices. State law, rules, and regulations govern the practice of nursing, while *Scope and Standards of Vascular Nursing Practice* guides nurses in the application of their professional skills and responsibilities.

Published by nursesbooks.org
The Publishing Program of ANA
American Nurses Association
600 Maryland Avenue, SW • Suite 100 West • Washington, DC 20024
1-800-274-4ANA • http://www.nursingworld.org/

ISBN 1-55810-221-3
04SSVN   2M   05/04

ACKNOWLEDGEMENTS

This document was developed by the Society for Vascular Nursing (SVN) Professional Education and Practice Committee. The members of the Committee gratefully acknowledge the work of others who initiated the original documents on vascular nursing practice and those who reviewed drafts of the document.

SVN Professional Education and Development Committee
Cathy Brown, BS, RN, RVT, CVN, RDCS, Co-Chair
Melinda Bullivant, BSN, RN, CVN, Co-Chair
Phyllis Gordon, MSN, RN, CS
Jeri Stevens, MS, MPH, RN, CS
Pamela Strecker, BSN, RN, CVN
Anne M. Aquila, MSN, RN,BC
Karen Hayden, MSN, RN
Kate York, MSN, RN, CNP
Michelle Baird, BSN, RN
Alison Cannon, MSN, RN
M. Kate Schmidt, BSN, RN, CVN, Board Liaison

SVN Staff Liaison
Belinda E. Puetz, PhD, RN
Patricia M. Adkison, MA

SVN Board of Directors, 2003–2004
Patricia A. Lewis, MSN, RN, CVN, President
Catherine Wiegand, MSN, RN, CNS, President Elect
Diane Treat-Jacobson, PhD, RN, Secretary
Carolyn Robinson, MSN, RN, CANP, CVN, Treasurer
M. Isobel Green, RN, CNS, CNC, CVN, Director
Anne M. Aquila, MSN, RN,BC, Director
Patricia A. Matula, MSN, RNNC, CCRN, CVN, Director
Rita C. Clark, BSN, RN, CVN, Director
Linda Ward, MS, RNC, CCRN, FNP-BC, Director

American Nurses Association (ANA) Staff
Carol J. Bickford, PhD, RN,BC, Content editor
Yvonne Humes, MSA
Winifred Carson-Smith, JD

CONTENTS

STANDARDS OF VASCULAR NURSING PRACTICE
STANDARDS OF CARE

STANDARD 1. ASSESSMENT
The vascular nurse collects patient health data to recognize and identify actual or potential vascular problems.

STANDARD 2. DIAGNOSIS
The vascular nurse analyzes the assessment data and, in conjunction with the patient, significant others, and interdisciplinary team, determine diagnoses.

STANDARD 3. OUTCOME IDENTIFICATION
The vascular nurse, in partnership with the patient, significant others, and the interdisciplinary team, identifies expected outcomes individualized to the patient's health status.

STANDARD 4. PLANNING
The vascular nurse promotes and supports the development of programs, policies, and services that provide interventions to improve the vascular health status of populations. The vascular nurse develops a plan of care that prescribes interventions to attain expected outcomes.

STANDARD 5. IMPLEMENTATION
The vascular nurse implements the interventions identified in the plan of care.

STANDARD 6. EVALUATION
The vascular nurse evaluates the patient's progress toward attainment of expected outcomes.

Standards of Vascular Nursing Practice
Standards of Professional Performance

STANDARD 1. QUALITY OF CARE
The vascular nurse systematically evaluates the quality of care and effectiveness of vascular nursing practice.

STANDARD 2. PERFORMANCE APPRAISAL
The vascular nurse evaluates one's own vascular nursing practice in relation to professional practice standards and relevant statutes and regulations.

STANDARD 3. EDUCATION
The vascular nurse acquires and maintains current knowledge and competency in nursing practice.

STANDARD 4. COLLEGIALITY
The vascular nurse interacts with, and contributes to the professional development of, peers and other healthcare providers as colleagues.

STANDARD 5. ETHICS
The vascular nurse's assessments, actions, and recommendations on behalf of patients are determined and implemented in an ethical manner.

STANDARD 6. COLLABORATION
The vascular nurse collaborates with the patient, significant others, and the interdisciplinary team in providing patient care.

STANDARD 7. RESEARCH
The vascular nurse uses research findings in practice to improve the quality of care for patients, and shares this knowledge with the interdisciplinary team.

STANDARD 8. RESOURCE UTILIZATION
The vascular nurse considers factors related to safety, effectiveness, and cost in planning and delivering patient care to maximize resources while maintaining quality of care.

Standards of Advanced Practice Vascular Nursing
Standards of Care

Standard 1. Assessment

The advanced practice vascular nurse collects comprehensive patient health data.

Standard 2. Diagnosis

The advanced practice vascular nurse critically analyzes the assessment data in determining the diagnoses.

Standard 3. Outcome Identification

The advanced practice vascular nurse identifies expected outcomes derived from the assessment data and diagnoses, and individualizes expected outcomes with the patient and with the healthcare team when appropriate.

Standard 4. Planning

The advanced practice vascular nurse develops a comprehensive plan of care that includes interventions and treatments to attain expected outcomes.

Standard 5. Implementation

The advanced practice vascular nurse prescribes, orders, or implements interventions and treatments identified for the plan of care.

Standard 5a. Case Management and Coordination of Care

The advanced practice vascular nurse provides comprehensive clinical coordination of care and case management.

Standard 5b. Consultation

The advanced practice vascular nurse provides consultation to influence the plan of care for patients, enhance the abilities of others, and effect change in the system.

Standard 5c. Health Promotion, Health Maintenance, and Health Teaching

The advanced practice vascular nurse employs complex strategies, interventions, and teaching to promote, maintain, and improve health and prevent illness and injury.

Standard 5d. Prescriptive Authority and Treatment

The advanced practice vascular nurse prescribes both pharmacologic and nonpharmacologic interventions, procedures, and treatments in accordance with state and federal laws and regulations to treat illness and improve functional health or to provide preventive care to patients with vascular disease.

Standard 5e. Referral

The advanced practice vascular nurse identifies the need for additional care and makes referrals as needed.

Standard 6. Evaluation

The advanced practice vascular nurse evaluates the patient's progress in attaining expected outcomes.

STANDARDS OF ADVANCED PRACTICE
VASCULAR NURSING
STANDARDS OF PROFESSIONAL PERFORMANCE

STANDARD 1. QUALITY OF CARE
The advanced practice vascular nurse develops criteria for and evaluates the quality of care and effectiveness of advanced practice vascular nursing.

STANDARD 2. SELF-EVALUATION
The advanced practice vascular nurse continuously evaluates one's own vascular nursing practice in relation to professional practice standards and relevant statutes and regulations, and is accountable to the public and to the profession for providing competent clinical care.

STANDARD 3. EDUCATION
The advanced practice vascular nurse acquires and maintains current knowledge and skills in the specialty area of vascular nursing.

STANDARD 4. LEADERSHIP
The advanced practice vascular nurse serves as a leader and role model for the professional development of peers, colleagues, and others.

STANDARD 5. ETHICS
The advanced practice vascular nurse integrates ethical principles and norms in all areas of practice.

STANDARD 6. INTERDISCIPLINARY PROCESS
The advanced practice vascular nurse promotes an interdisciplinary process in providing patient care.

STANDARD 7. RESEARCH
The advanced practice vascular nurse uses research findings to discover, examine, and evaluate knowledge, theories, and creative approaches to healthcare practices.

INTRODUCTION

The Society for Vascular Nursing (SVN), an international association, was founded in 1982 for the purpose of promoting excellence in the compassionate and comprehensive management of individuals and their families who suffer from vascular disease. SVN members, the Board, and expert consultants facilitated the development of this document. Its purpose is to define the patient population, to provide a framework for professional growth and development for vascular nurses, and to outline the scope of practice and standards of vascular nursing care for vascular nurses.

The years since the founding of SVN have been characterized by significant changes in health care and the associated sciences and evolving research, resulting in new thinking about the causes, treatment and prevention of vascular disease. This international association and its members continue to lead in addressing these changes and patient needs.

To help the profession and the public better understand the practice of vascular nursing and thereby value today's vascular nurses, the Society for Vascular Nursing supported and charged a task force to examine historical documents, references and resources and then create the nursing specialty's first scope and standards of practice. The purpose of this resulting document is to define the patient population, to provide a framework for professional growth and development for vascular nurses, and to outline the scope of practice and standards of vascular nursing care.

The scope of practice statement defines vascular disease, but more importantly serves to emphasize the unique practice characteristics of the vascular nurse moving beyond pathophysiology and diagnosis to identify and treat human responses to actual or potential alterations in vascular system function. Vascular nurses today focus their emphasis on the promotion of health, assessment for alterations of function, and implementation of strategies to assist individuals to maintain, regain or improve function and prevent disability. Discussion of the practice environments and educational preparation of the vascular nurse generalist and the advanced practice vascular nurse identify those behaviors, responsibilities, functions and skills that involve a specific and unique body of knowledge. The scope statement provides answers to the who, what, where, when, why, and how questions about this nursing specialty.

As a complement, the standards for vascular nursing practice are generic statements that define the responsibilities and accountability to the profession and the public of all registered nurses who care for patients with vascular disease. These standards reflect the values and priorities of the profession of nursing as they relate to the specialty of vascular nursing and provide directives and a measurement framework for minimal levels of nursing practice in the care of vascular patients in any setting. These standards are listed are the next two pages and delineated with their respective measurement criteria starting on page 13.

The specialty scope and standards of practice must be considered in relation to the definition of nursing, *Code of Ethics for Nurses with Interpretive Statements* (2001), and *Nursing's Social Policy Statement, 2nd Edition* (2003) and must be reviewed and revised on a regular basis to reflect changes in health care and the nursing profession. In 2004 *Scope and Standards of Vascular Nursing* completed the American Nurses Association's established review and recognition process for specialty nursing scope and standards of practice.

The evolving nature of vascular nursing is a reflection of technological advances, greater scientific understanding, and a growing research base. Nursing has moved from an era of needing only to provide good, safe, care to the patient with vascular dysfunction to the present era of incorporation of science and research into practice. Given rapid changes in healthcare delivery trends and technologies, the task of defining the scope of vascular nursing is complex. This document is intended to be both futuristic and flexible in nature, allowing for the response to emerging issues and technologies in the delivery of health care as well as in the practice of vascular nursing.

SCOPE OF VASCULAR NURSING PRACTICE

Vascular nursing is a unique area within the nursing discipline that specializes in the care of individuals who have known or predicted physiological alterations of the vascular system. Vascular nursing promotes and protects the health of individuals, and seeks to educate individuals and their families at risk for vascular disease using knowledge from the fields of nursing, medicine, and the social sciences. The practice of vascular nursing is dynamic in response to the needs of individuals with vascular disease, as well as to advancements in the fields of vascular medicine, interventional radiology and vascular surgery. Its focus includes health promotion, assessment for alterations of function, and implementation of strategies to assist patients to maintain, regain, or improve function and prevent disability. Potential recipients of vascular nursing care are individuals with vascular system dysfunction, their families and significant others, and the society in which they live.

Vascular Disease Defined

Vascular disease encompasses a wide array of arterial, venous, and lymphatic problems and may be acute or chronic in nature. The epidemiology of vascular disease provides an overview of the magnitude of the disease and serves to define the patient population. Major categories of disease that produce alterations of concern to vascular nurses include cerebrovascular disease, aneurysmal disease, peripheral arterial occlusive disease, acute arterial disease, venous disease, lymphatic disease, vascular trauma, congenital vascular conditions, nonatherosclerotic arterial disease, wound management, pain, and diabetes mellitus. Vascular nursing care is provided to patients of all ages across the continuum of care from acute care to community care.

Arterial Disease

Causes of arterial disease are extremely varied; however, atherosclerosis is the underlying mechanism responsible for peripheral arterial disease (PAD). PAD encompasses those entities that result in arterial occlusions in vessels other than those of the coronary and intracranial vascular beds. Although PAD includes the extracranial, carotid, upper extremity, visceral, and renal circulation, the term is usually applied to disease involving the circulation of the lower extremities (Ouriel, 2001). Among those with lower extremity PAD, approximately two-thirds are asymptomatic (Hiatt & Cooke, 2001). It is important to identify these patients since PAD is a marker of generalized atherosclerosis, thereby placing the individual at increased risk of concomitant coronary and cerebrovascular disease (Treat-Jacobson & Walsh, 2003).

Individuals with lower extremity PAD often present for treatment because of symptoms of intermittent claudication or critical limb ischemia. Critical limb ischemia may take the form of rest pain, minor tissue loss (ulceration), or gangrene. The prevalence of PAD increases dramatically with age, from only 3% for ages 40 to 59 to nearly 20% for those ages 70 or above (Hackam & Anand, 2003). The aging of the baby boom generation and increasing life span yield a projected 40% increase in the total number of Americans with PAD by the year 2020 (Hackam & Anand, 2003; Criqui, Langer & Fronek, 1992). Those with PAD are at significantly increased risk of death from myocardial infarction and stroke. It accounts for nearly three-fourths of all deaths from cardiovascular disease (American Heart Association, 1999). Major risk factors for PAD include male gender, advanced age (> 50 years), diabetes mellitus, tobacco use, sedentary life style, uncontrolled hypertension, and dyslipidemia.

The focus now on the prevention of vascular disease provides generalist and advanced practice vascular nurses with a new opportunity to enhance patient care. All patients presenting for treatment of their extremity should have their risk factors rigorously assessed, and appropriate therapies instituted to decrease the risks of both peripheral progression and cardiovascular mortality.

Diabetes mellitus deserves special consideration, since 18.2 million people or 6.3% of the total US population have diabetes. Of those age 60 years or older, 8.6 million or 18.3% of all people in this age group have diabetes (National Diabetes Information Clearinghouse, 2002). Diabetes accelerates the clinical course of atherosclerosis in three vascular beds: lower extremity arteries, coronary arteries, and extracranial carotid arteries (Beckman, Creager & Libby, 2003; Canto & Iskandrian, 2003).

Epidemiological evidence confirms the relationship between diabetes and increased presence of lower extremity PAD. Individuals commonly develop symptomatic forms of PAD, intermittent claudication, and amputation. According to the Framingham study, the presence of diabetes increased the risk of claudication by 250% in men and 760% in women (Hackam & Anand, 2003). In addition, patients with diabetes and lower extremity PAD may experience diminished sensation due to diabetic neuropathy, and a decreased resistance to infection in poorly controlled diabetes accounts for the high incidence of gangrenous changes of the feet. Unfortunately, more than 60% of nontraumatic lower-limb amputations in the US occur among people with diabetes. In 2000–2001, approximately 82,000 nontraumatic lower-limb amputations were performed per year among people with diabetes. Heart disease is the leading cause of diabetes-related deaths (65%) and a 2 to 4 times higher risk of stroke exists in individuals with diabetes (National Diabetes Information Clearinghouse, 2004).

Abnormal metabolic states that accompany diabetes alter arterial function. Abnormalities include chronic hyperglycemia, dyslipidemia, and insulin resistance. These conditions increase the arteries' susceptibility to atherosclerosis. Diabetes then alters the function of cell types including the endothelium, platelets, and smooth muscles resulting in ultimate vascular dysfunction (Beckman et al, 2003).

The effects of diabetes are multiple. Vascular nurses are in a prime position to educate the individual with diabetes about the disease process and the relationship of diabetes to cardiac and vascular disease. Better diabetes management can influence cardiac and vascular function. Vascular nurse generalists and specialists work together to meet the needs of this patient population. Ideally, blood sugar should be normalized in the diabetic patient before an intervention. For the advanced practice vascular nurse, this may involve switching the patient from oral agents to insulin, and subsequent monitoring for glycemic control.

Control of sepsis in the diabetic foot may help control hyperglycemia and ketoacidosis. This involves appropriate use of antibiotics, judicious wound care, and monitoring for complications. Generalist and advanced practice vascular nurses can work collaboratively to institute measures aimed at the prevention and management of diabetic foot ulcers. In addition, education is aimed at teaching the diabetic patient ways to reduce the risk of limb amputation, including daily foot assessment, attention to foot hygiene, and foot protection such as proper footwear.

As the population ages, abdominal aortic aneurysms (AAAs) are an increasing healthcare concern in the Unites States today because the incidence and prevalence increases with age. It is estimated that 1.5 million people in the United States are living with AAAs, with 200,000 new cases diagnosed yearly (Makary, 2001). In the United States, half of all patients with untreated AAAs die of an aortic rupture within five years. AAAs are the nation's 13th leading cause of death, killing close to 17,000 Americans each year (Gillum,1995). Men are four times as likely as women to develop an AAA. Male gender and smoking are the strongest risk factors for AAA (Verloes, Sakalihasan, Koulischer & Limet, 1995). 75% of those diagnosed with AAAs will be asymptomatic (Mitchell, Rutherford, & Krupski, 1999). For most of these patients, management is directed toward early detection and appropriate surgical intervention by preventing aneurysm rupture. Vascular nurses must be familiar with this disease process to effectively counsel and educate patients and their families regarding aneurysm detection and treatment options.

Cerebrovascular disease dramatically affects the lives of millions of Americans, their families, communities in which they reside, healthcare delivery systems treating those affected, health promotion organizations fighting the battle against stroke, and health policy makers who influence the national agenda. Stroke ranks third among causes of death in the United States. It is estimated that more than 700,000 incident strokes occur every year, adding to the number of approximately 4.7 million stroke survivors (American Stroke Association & JCAHO Collaborate, 2003). Stroke is the leading cause of serious, long-term disability. Vascular nurses provide education to patients regarding stroke risk and warning signs, thereby assisting in early patient recognition and prompt treatment of a cerebrovascular event such as a transient ischemic attack (TIA) or evolving stroke.

Vascular nurses may choose to focus their practice on the care of individuals requiring surgical or interventional strategies such as to carotid artery surgery, lower extremity revascularization by either surgical or endovascular approaches, surgery for aneurysmal disease, renal/mesenteric disease, limb amputation, and the creation of vascular access for hemodialysis to manage their arterial problems.

Non-atherosclerotic Arterial Disease

Non-atherosclerotic arterial diseases include but are not limited to Buerger's disease, Raynaud's syndrome, fibromuscular dysplasia, trauma, compartment syndrome, arterial infection, compression syndromes, congenital conditions, and hyperviscosity syndromes.

Venous Disease

Venous disease encompasses a wide spectrum of disorders, ranging from those with benign, primarily cosmetic concerns, such as spider telangiectasias and superficial varicose veins, to those with potentially life- or limb-threatening consequences, such as acute deep vein thrombosis and pulmonary emboli. Other manifestations of venous pathology include superficial venous thrombophlebitis, variceal bleeding, and chronic venous insufficiency (CVI).

An estimated 500,000 to 600,000 people in the United States have CVI, which is the most common venous disorder. The term CVI refers to a constellation of limb symptoms including edema, pain, pigmentation changes, and disability, which can progress to chronic ulceration. CVI is responsible for 90% of lower extremity ulcerations. (de Araujo, Valencia, Federman & Kirsner, 2003).

The advanced practice vascular nurse who is an expert in venous ulcer care may provide supervision or direction for ulcer management (topical agents, dressing techniques), assist with the implementation of medical therapies when appropriate, and provide patient education and support.

Lymphatic Disease

The lymphatic system consists of an extensive network that collects lymph from the various organs and tissues and connects to an elaborate system of collecting vessels that transport the lymph to the blood stream. Lymphedema results from a malformation or obstruction of the lymphatic vessels or nodes. Lymphedema may be acquired or congenital, and it often develops secondary to another event, such as trauma, or surgical intervention, such as mastectomy.

The advanced practice vascular nurse may play a role in the differential diagnosis of lymphedema through history taking and a comprehensive physical examination. Both generalist and advanced practice vascular nursing interventions are aimed at reducing edema, maintaining the edema-free state, control of infection, and providing education and emotional support.

Practice Characteristics

Vascular nurses move beyond the diagnosis of pathophysiology to identifying and treating human responses to actual or potential health problems related to phenomena affected by vascular system dysfunction. Specific phenomena that form a framework for vascular nursing practice include:

- *Consciousness*—The awareness of and interaction with the surrounding environment as well as the higher thought processes; alterations include problems such as TIAs and stroke.

- *Circulation*—The ability to maintain adequate blood flow/perfusion to the brain, extremities, and vital organs; alterations include stroke, acute and chronic upper and lower extremity arterial and venous disease, ulcerations, gangrene, and amputation.

- *Rest/Sleep*—Behaviors needed for restorative function, rest needed to promote healing and to maintain an overall sense of well-being.

- *Sensation*—The ability to sense and distinguish internal and external stimuli; alterations include decreased sensation related to diabetic neuropathy and pain related to the overall mechanisms for arterial, venous, and lymphatic diseases.

- *Activity*—The ability to move freely within the environment; alterations include stroke, chronic limb ischemia, gangrene, and amputation.

- *Skin Integrity*—The maintenance of intact skin, without breakdown; alterations include arterial, venous, and diabetic ulcers.

- *Adequate Nutrition*—The balance of nutrients to maintain health including an overall sense of well-being, the healing of surgical wounds, and the healing of lower extremity vascular wounds.

- *Response to illness/coping*—The ability to form and maintain social support and relationships; alterations include social isolation and role changes secondary to vascular system disease.

- *Self-care*—The ability to provide one's basic needs; alterations include the inability to care for one's self.

Vascular nurses rely on a specialized body of knowledge, skills, technology, and experience to respond and adapt to patient need. Vascular nurses use the nursing process to deliver care including assessment, diagnosis, outcome identification, planning, implementation, and evaluation. Vascular nursing practice is characterized by interventions that promote health, assess for alterations in function, assist patients to regain or improve their function, and prevent further disability.

Promotion of Health

The vascular nurse stresses health promotion, reflecting nursing's longstanding commitment to the well-being of the individual, family, group, and community. The vascular nurse performs assessments, targets individuals at risk for vascular disease, and initiates interventions aimed at promoting or maintaining vascular health.

The focus now on prevention of vascular disease provides generalist and advanced practice vascular nurses with a new opportunity to influence patient care. Vascular nurses are in a prime position to educate the individual with vascular disease regarding the disease process, thereby decreasing the risk of poor outcomes such as stroke, formation of vascular wounds, and limb loss. Vascular nurses must be familiar with the disease process to effectively counsel and educate patients and their families regarding treatment options.

All patients presenting for treatment of their vascular problem should have their risk factors rigorously assessed, and appropriate therapies instituted to decrease the risks of both progression of vascular complications and cardiovascular mortality. Vascular nurses practicing in a variety of inpatient and outpatient settings can assist patients with risk factor modification. They can help patients stop smoking, maintain glycemic control, normalize high blood pressure and lipid levels, maintain anti-platelet therapy, and foster participation in exercise programs, thereby promoting positive patient outcomes.

Assessment for Alterations in Function

The vascular nurse performs assessments and collects data regarding the health status of the individual with vascular disease in a systematic and ongoing manner. Collected data include not only the physical needs of the individual but the psychosocial and spiritual needs as well. Out of data collection, nursing diagnoses are formulated, measurable goals are determined, and a plan of care developed, implemented, and evaluated. Information obtained from the individuals or family is communicated to other members of the care team.

Measures to Maintain, Regain, or Improve Function and Prevent Disability

A major focus of clinical vascular nursing care involves teaching the individual or family ways to maintain, regain, or to improve function, as well as to prevent disability. These include information relative to the individual's specific vascular problem as well as instruction on health-promoting behaviors including but not limited to diet, exercise, blood glucose control/monitoring, smoking cessation, and hypertension management. Teaching must take into consideration the capabilities and limitations of the individual or family and collaboration with other professionals and specialists such as dietitians. Vascular nurses may also focus on the overall assessment, treatment, and evaluation of individuals requiring surgical or interventional strategies to manage their arterial problem.

Practice Environments, Education, and Roles

The Vascular Nurse Generalist

Registered nurses at the generalist level have completed a nursing program and met state licensure examination requirements. Registered nurses who practice in vascular nursing settings may work as staff nurses, case managers, nurse managers, and in other roles in the field of vascular nursing. In today's dynamic healthcare environment, vascular nurse generalists practice in a variety of settings. These settings vary in purpose, type, location, acuity, and the auspices under which they operate. Practice settings include, but are not limited to, acute and subacute care facilities, home care agencies, ambulatory care clinics, outpatient service facilities, residential facilities, skilled nursing facilities, private practices, physicians' offices, and wound care clinics. Educational preparation for the vascular nurse generalist ranges from a two-year associate degree to a four-year baccalaureate degree.

The Advanced Practice Vascular Nurse

The advanced practice registered nurse in vascular nursing is a licensed registered nurse who is educationally prepared as a clinical nurse specialist or a nurse practitioner with at least the master's degree level. Advanced practice vascular nurses have acquired in-depth knowledge and clinical skills to prepare them for expansion and advancement in vascular nursing practice. Consistent with a broadened knowledge base, advanced practice vascular nursing is characterized by increased complexity of clinical decision-making related to the assessment and management of individuals with vascular disease, as well as greater skill in managing organizations and environments.

Nurses in advanced practice vascular nursing roles may provide comprehensive physical assessment and demonstrate a high level of autonomy and expert skill in the diagnosis and treatment of the complex responses of individuals, families, or communities to actual or potential health problems. They formulate clinical decisions to manage acute and chronic illness and promote wellness. They provide and deliver health care that is accessible to patients in various settings and throughout the life cycle.

Advanced practice vascular nurses integrate education, research, management, leadership, and consultation into clinical roles. They function in collegial relationships with nursing peers and other professionals and people who influence the healthcare environment in many diverse settings. By virtue of this integration, advanced practice vascular nurses are clinicians, educators, researchers, and administrators. Specific tasks will be influenced by the care setting and the role of the nurse. Emphasis on specific elements of the nursing process — assessment, diagnosis, planning, intervention, and evaluation — will vary with the role as well as setting.

Clinically focused tasks performed by the advanced practice vascular nurse might include:

- Diagnosis and management of vascular wounds
- Performance of preoperative/preprocedural history and physical examinations
- Postoperative management
- Use of ultrasound equipment for testing
- First assistant in the operating room or radiology suite
- Management of an anticoagulation clinic
- Membership on a stroke team
- Dialysis access evaluation
- Use of telemedicine for home care management or house calls to homebound vascular patients.

Administrative tasks include data collection and outcomes management and evaluation, protocol development, and staff management. Research activities include the design and implementation of research projects, data collection and analysis, publication of findings, and patient management during research projects.

The advanced practice vascular nurse is responsible for identifying the scope of practice permitted by state and federal laws and regulations, the professional code of ethics, and the professional practice standards. In addition, his or her experience, education, knowledge, and abilities circumscribe the nurse's competence (American Nurses Association, 1996).

Certification

Certification is the process by which the American Nurses Credentialing Center (ANCC) Boards on Certification (BOCs) validate, based on predetermined standards, an individual's knowledge, skills, and abilities on a defined functional and clinical area of nursing practice. The Cardiac/Vascular Nurse certification examination is now available to those nurses providing nursing care to individuals with diagnosed cardiac/vascular disease as well as those identified at risk for cardiac/vascular events (American Nurses Credentialing Center, 2001).

Ethics

The practice of the generalist and advanced practice vascular nurse is guided by *Code of Ethics for Nurses with Interpretive Statements* (American Nurses Association, 2001). The vascular nurse following this professional code acknowledges the patient's rights to privacy and confidentiality, to be informed, and to be treated with dignity. The vascular nurse recognizes the patient not only as a unique individual, but also as part of a broader structure encompassing family or other significant relationships. The generalist and advanced practice vascular nurse acknowledges the patient's cultural beliefs, diversity, and individual uniqueness, and ensures that vascular nursing care is non-judgmental and non-discriminatory. The vascular nurse serves as a patient advocate, works to facilitate patient decision-making, promotes an ethical practice environment, and promotes professional integrity.

In addition, the advanced practice vascular nurse acknowledges the patient's rights to information, self-determination, and truthful disclosure. The advanced practice vascular nurse considers the patient's cultural beliefs, diversity, and individual uniqueness when diagnosing, prescribing, and planning therapeutic interventions.

Future Considerations

The evolving nature of vascular nursing is a reflection of technological advances, greater scientific understanding, and a growing research base. Nursing has moved from an era of needing only to provide good, safe care to the patient with vascular dysfunction to the present era of incorporating science and research into care. Examples of this are the early treatment of stroke with thrombolytic agents and endovascular repair of aortic aneurysms.

Vascular nurses are increasingly involved in research activities as independent or collaborative researchers. Complementary medicine and alternative therapies are further expanding healthcare options, challenging vascular nurses to remain knowledgeable of developments so they are able to guide their patients in their use.

A major impact on the scope of practice in vascular nursing is the changing healthcare delivery system. Societal, economic, and political pressures are driving the development of less costly ways to meet the healthcare needs of consumers. Vascular nurses can be intimately involved in this process by using nurse specialists to deliver care. Advanced practice nurses, with their expanded body of knowledge and skills, can provide high-quality care in a more cost-effective manner. Examples of this might be a nurse-managed wound clinic or a nurse-run anticoagulation service. These advanced practice nurses can also function as consultants to other nurses and other healthcare team members. Collaboration, along with effective use of resources, cost containment, increased participation by recipients of care, timely achievement of goals, and continuity of care are concepts critical to the future of vascular nursing as well as other healthcare systems.

Professional Organization Goals and Direction

Vascular nurses are strongly encouraged to become active members of the Society for Vascular Nursing (SVN), a specialty nursing organization focused on provision of support services for the nurse providing care to individuals with vascular disease. This is accomplished through educational offerings, collaboration with fellow vascular nurses, maintenance of a web site for information and links to related organizations, grant funding for vascular nursing research, and recognition of achievement in the field of vascular nursing. The society produces a peer-reviewed professional nursing journal, *The Journal of Vascular Nursing*, which offers continuing education credits for selected articles. SVN holds an annual convention that serves as a forum for conducting the business of the society as well as for academic presentations and mentorship.

A secondary focus of the society is participation in primary disease prevention. SVN collaborates with other organizations, such as the Vascular Disease Foundation, to develop a national public campaign for peripheral arterial disease awareness. Patient education materials for risk factor reduction have been developed, as well as alliances with other nursing organizations that share similar concerns (e.g., smoking cessation). Members have developed a research priority agenda to promote nursing research for primary and secondary prevention of vascular disease.

SVN is a member of the Nursing Organization Alliance, which is actively involved with the ANA Agenda for the Future task force, and is a member of the Vascular Disease Foundation. The organization is interested in affecting the direction of both vascular nursing and public policy regarding atherosclerosis prevention and management.

Standards of Vascular Nursing Practice
Standards of Care

Standard 1. Assessment

The vascular nurse collects patient health data to recognize and identify actual or potential vascular problems.

Measurement Criteria

1. Data collection involves the patient, significant others, and the interdisciplinary team as appropriate.

2. The priority of data collection activities is determined by the patient's immediate condition or needs.

3. Pertinent data are collected using appropriate assessment techniques and instruments. Sources of assessment data can include not only the patient, but also family, social network, other healthcare clinicians, past and current medical records, and community agencies and systems (with consideration of the patient's confidentiality).

4. Relevant data derived from the nursing assessment are documented in a retrievable form.

5. The data collection process is systematic and ongoing.

STANDARD 2. DIAGNOSIS

The vascular nurse analyzes the assessment data and, in conjunction with the patient, significant others, and interdisciplinary team, determine diagnoses.

Measurement Criteria

1. Diagnoses are derived from the assessment data.

2. Diagnoses and vascular risk factors are discussed and validated with the patient, significant others, and the interdisciplinary team.

3. Diagnoses are documented in a manner that facilitates the identification of patient outcomes and their use in the plan of care and research.

4. Priorities are selected in partnership with the patient, significant others, and the interdisciplinary team.

STANDARD 3. OUTCOME IDENTIFICATION

The vascular nurse, in partnership with the patient, significant others, and the interdisciplinary team, identifies expected outcomes individualized to the patient's health status.

Measurement Criteria

1. Expected outcomes are derived from the diagnoses and reflect current scientific knowledge in vascular care and treatment.

2. Expected outcomes are mutually formulated with the patient, significant others, and the interdisciplinary team and are patient-oriented, evidence-based, realistic, attainable and cost-effective.

3. Expected outcomes are culturally appropriate and realistic in relation to the patient's present and potential capabilities and quality of life.

4. Expected outcomes are identified with consideration of the associated benefits and costs.

5. Expected outcomes are clearly stated and include a time estimate for attainment.

6. Expected outcomes provide direction for continuity of care.

7. Expected outcomes are documented as measurable goals and shared with the interdisciplinary team.

STANDARD 4. PLANNING

The vascular nurse promotes and supports the development of programs, policies, and services that provide interventions to improve the vascular health status of populations. The vascular nurse develops a plan of care that prescribes interventions to attain expected outcomes.

Measurement Criteria

1. The vascular plan of care is individualized to the patient (e.g., age-appropriate, culturally sensitive) and the patient's condition or needs:

    • Identifies priorities of care in relation to expected outcomes.

    • Identifies effective interventions to achieve outcomes.

    • Specifies evidence-based interventions that reflect current best practices and research.

    • Reflects the patient's motivation, health beliefs, and functional capabilities.

    • Includes an educational program related to the patient's health problems, risk reduction, self-care activities, and quality of life.

    • Indicates responsibilities of the nurse, the patient, the family and other significant persons, and the interdisciplinary team members in implementing the plan.

    • Gives direction to the patient care activities that are designated by the nurse for the patient, significant others and the interdisciplinary teams.

    • Provides the appropriate referral and case management to ensure continuity of care.

    • Considers the benefits and costs of interventions in relation to outcomes.

2. The plan is developed with the patient, significant others, and the interdisciplinary team, and identifies evidence-based interventions to attain expected outcomes.

3. The plan reflects current vascular nursing practice.

4. Priorities for care are established.

5. The plan is documented in a format that allows modification, as necessary, interdisciplinary access to its information, and retrieval of data for analysis and research.

STANDARD 5. IMPLEMENTATION

The vascular nurse implements the interventions identified in the plan of care.

Measurement Criteria

1. Interventions are implemented according to the established plan of care.

2. Interventions are evidence-based.

3. Interventions are implemented in a safe, timely, ethical, and appropriate manner.

4. Interventions are performed according to the vascular nurse's level of education and practice.

5. Interventions are modified based on continued assessment of the patient's response to treatment and other clinical indicators of effectiveness.

6. Interventions are documented in a format that is related to patient outcomes, accessible to the interdisciplinary team, and retrievable for future analysis and research.

STANDARD 6. EVALUATION

The vascular nurse evaluates the patient's progress toward attainment of expected outcomes.

Measurement Criteria

1. Evaluation is systematic, ongoing, and criterion-based.

2. The patient, significant others, and the interdisciplinary team are involved in the evaluation process, as appropriate, to ascertain the patient's level of satisfaction with care and to evaluate the benefits and cost associated with the treatment process.

3. Ongoing assessment data are used to revise diagnoses, outcomes, and the plan of care, as needed.

4. Revisions in diagnoses, outcomes, and the plan of care are documented.

5. The effectiveness of interventions is evaluated in relation to outcomes.

6. The patient's responses to interventions are documented in a format that is related to expected outcomes, accessible to the interdisciplinary team, and retrievable for analysis and future research.

STANDARDS OF PROFESSIONAL PERFORMANCE

STANDARD 1. QUALITY OF CARE

The vascular nurse systematically evaluates the quality of care and effectiveness of vascular nursing practice.

Measurement Criteria

The vascular nurse:

1. Participates in quality-of-care activities as appropriate to the nurse's education, position, and practice environment. Such activities may include:

    *   Identification of aspects of care important for quality monitoring; for example, risk factor analysis, symptom management, follow-up post procedures, patient satisfaction, and quality of life.

    *   Analysis of quality data to identify opportunities for improving vascular nursing care.

    *   Development of policies, procedures, and practice guidelines to improve quality of vascular care .

    *   Utilization of existing, or development of new, quality indicators used to monitor the effectiveness of vascular nursing care.

    *   Collection of data to monitor quality and effectiveness of vascular nursing care.

    *   Formulation of recommendations to improve vascular nursing practice or patient outcomes.

    *   Implementation of activities to enhance the quality of vascular nursing practice.

    *   Participation on interdisciplinary teams to evaluate clinical practice or health services.

2. Seeks feedback from the patient and significant others about the quality and outcome of the patient's care.

3. Uses the results of quality-of-care activities to initiate changes throughout the healthcare delivery system, as appropriate.

STANDARD 2. PERFORMANCE APPRAISAL

The vascular nurse evaluates one's own vascular nursing practice in relation to professional practice standards and relevant statutes and regulations.

Measurement Criteria

The vascular nurse:

1. Engages in performance appraisal of one's own clinical practice and role performance on a regular basis, identifying areas of strength as well as areas where professional development would be beneficial.

2. Seeks constructive feedback regarding one's own practice from peers, professional colleagues, patients, and others.

3. Takes action to achieve goals identified during performance appraisal and peer review, resulting in changes in practice and role performance.

4. Participates in peer review activities.

5. Practices in a manner that reflects knowledge of current professional practice standards, laws, and regulations.

STANDARD 3. EDUCATION

The vascular nurse acquires and maintains current knowledge and competency in nursing practice.

Measurement Criteria

The vascular nurse:

1. Participates in professional development to improve clinical knowledge, enhance role performance, and increase knowledge of professional issues.

2. Seeks experiences and independent learning that reflect current clinical practice in order to maintain current clinical skills and experience.

3. Acquires additional knowledge and skills appropriate to the specialty area and practice setting by participating in educational programs, conferences, workshops, and interdisciplinary professional meetings.

STANDARD 4. COLLEGIALITY

The vascular nurse interacts with, and contributes, to the professional development of, peers and other healthcare providers as colleagues.

Measurement Criteria

The vascular nurse:

1. Uses opportunities in practice to exchange knowledge, skills, and clinical observation with colleagues and others.

2. Provides peers with constructive feedback regarding their practice.

3. Interacts with colleagues to enhance their own professional nursing practice and promote interdisciplinary collaboration.

4. Contributes to an environment that is conducive to the clinical education of nursing students, other healthcare students, and other employees, as appropriate.

5. Contributes to a supportive and healthy work environment.

STANDARD 5. ETHICS

The vascular nurse's assessments, actions, and recommendations on behalf of patients are determined and implemented in an ethical manner.

Measurement Criteria

The vascular nurse:

1. Is guided in practice by *Code of Ethics for Nurses with Interpretive Statements* (American Nurses Association, 2001).

2. Maintains patient confidentiality within ethical, legal, and regulatory parameters.

3. Acts as a patient advocate and assists patients in developing the skills to advocate for themselves.

4. Delivers care in a nonjudgmental and nondiscriminatory manner that is sensitive to patient diversity, maintaining a professional relationship with patients at all times.

5. Delivers care in a manner that preserves patient autonomy, dignity, and rights.

6. Strives to prevent ethical problems, and uses available resources in formulating ethical decisions.

Standard 6. Collaboration

The vascular nurse collaborates with the patient, significant others, and the interdisciplinary team in providing patient care.

Measurement Criteria

The vascular nurse:

1. Communicates with the patient, significant others, and the interdisciplinary team regarding patient care and the vascular nurse's role in the provision of care.

2. Collaborates with the patient, significant others, and the interdisciplinary team in the formulation of overall goals, plans, and decisions related to patient care and the delivery of vascular services.

3. Consults with other healthcare providers for patient care, as needed.

4. Makes referrals, including provisions for continuity of care, as needed.

5. Collaborates with other disciplines in teaching, consultation, management, and research.

STANDARD 7. RESEARCH

The vascular nurse uses research findings in practice to improve the quality of care for patients, and shares this knowledge with the interdisciplinary team.

Measurement Criteria

The vascular nurse:

1. Uses the best available evidence, preferably research data, to develop the patient's plan of care, vascular interventions, and expected outcomes.

2. Participates in research as appropriate to their education, position, and practice environment. This may include:

    • Identifying clinical problems suitable for vascular nursing research.

    • Participating in data collection.

    • Participating in unit, organization, or community research committees or programs.

    • Sharing research findings with others through discussion groups, professional presentations, and publications.

    • Conducting research as an individual investigator or as a member of a research team according to education and experience.

    • Critiquing research for application to clinical practice.

    • Using research findings in the development of policies, procedures, and practice guidelines for patient care.

    • Consulting with research colleagues and experts.

3. Participates in clinical trials and human subject protection activities as appropriate, recognizing the vulnerability of subjects in the research study.

STANDARD 8. RESOURCE UTILIZATION

The vascular nurse considers factors related to safety, effectiveness, and cost in planning and delivering patient care to maximize resources while maintaining quality of care.

Measurement Criteria

The vascular nurse:

1. Evaluates factors related to safety, effectiveness, availability, and cost when choosing between practice options that would result in the same expected patient outcome.

2. Assists the patient and significant others in identifying and securing appropriate and available services to address vascular health-related needs.

3. Refers, assigns, or delegates patient care activities as defined by the state nurse practice acts and according to the knowledge and skills of the designated caregiver.

4. Refers, assigns, or delegates patient care activities based on the whole needs and condition of the patient, the potential for harm, the stability of the patient's condition, the complexity of the task, and the predictability of the outcome.

5. Assists the patient and significant others in becoming consumers informed about the cost, risk, and benefits of vascular treatment and care.

STANDARDS OF ADVANCED VASCULAR NURSING PRACTICE
STANDARDS OF CARE

The advanced practice vascular nurse is expected to meet the previous standards and measurement criteria as well as those specific to advanced practice.

STANDARD 1. ASSESSMENT

The advanced practice vascular nurse collects comprehensive patient health data.

Measurement Criteria

1. Assessment techniques are based on research and knowledge.

2. Diagnostic tests and procedures relevant to the patient's current status are initiated as indicated and are interpreted.

STANDARD 2. DIAGNOSIS

The advanced practice vascular nurse critically analyzes the assessment data in determining the diagnoses.

Measurement Criteria

1. Diagnoses are derived and prioritized from the assessment data using appropriate complex clinical reasoning.

2. A differential diagnosis is formulated by systematically comparing and contrasting clinical findings.

3. Diagnoses are made using advanced synthesis of information obtained during the interview, physical examination, diagnostic tests, or diagnostic procedures.

STANDARD 3. OUTCOME IDENTIFICATION

The advanced practice vascular nurse identifies expected outcomes derived from the assessment data and diagnoses, and individualizes expected outcomes with the patient and with the healthcare team when appropriate.

Measurement Criteria

1. Expected outcomes are identified with consideration of the associated risk, benefits, and costs.

2. Expected outcomes are consistent with current scientific and clinical practice knowledge.

3. Expected outcomes are modified based on changes in the patient's healthcare status.

STANDARD 4. PLANNING

The advanced practice vascular nurse develops a comprehensive plan of care that includes interventions and treatments to attain expected outcomes.

Measurement Criteria

1. The comprehensive plan of care describes the assessment/diagnostic strategies and therapeutic interventions that reflect current healthcare knowledge, research, and practice.

2. The comprehensive plan of care reflects the responsibilities of the advanced practice vascular nurse and the patient, and may include delegation of responsibilities to others.

3. The comprehensive plan of care addresses strategies for promotion and restoration of health and prevention of illness, injury, and disease through independent clinical decision-making.

4. The comprehensive plan of care is documented and modified to provide direction to other members of the healthcare team.

STANDARD 5. IMPLEMENTATION

The advanced practice vascular nurse prescribes, orders, or implements interventions and treatments identified for the plan of care.

Measurement Criteria

1. Interventions and treatments are performed or implemented with knowledge of healthcare research findings and based on scientific theory.

2. Interventions and treatments are performed within the scope of advanced practice nursing.

STANDARD 5A. CASE MANAGEMENT AND COORDINATION OF CARE

The advanced practice vascular nurse provides comprehensive clinical coordination of care and case management.

Measurement Criteria

1. Case management and clinical coordination of care services are provided using sophisticated data synthesis with consideration of the patient's complex needs and desired outcomes. This results in integration of health care that is accessible, available, high quality, and cost-effective.

2. Health-related services and additional specialized care are negotiated with the patient and appropriate systems, agencies, and providers.

STANDARD 5B. CONSULTATION

The advanced practice vascular nurse provides consultation to influence the plan of care for patients, enhance the abilities of others, and effect change in the system.

Measurement Criteria

1. Consultation activities are based upon theoretical frameworks.

2. Consultation is based upon mutual respect, and defined role responsibilities are established with the patient.

3. Consultation recommendations are communicated in terms that facilitate understanding and involve the patient in decision-making.

4. The decision to implement the system change or plan of care remains the responsibility of the patient.

STANDARD 5C. HEALTH PROMOTION, HEALTH MAINTENANCE, AND HEALTH TEACHING

The advanced practice vascular nurse employs complex strategies, interventions, and teaching to promote, maintain, and improve health and prevent illness and injury.

Measurement Criteria

1. Strategies for health promotion and disease, illness, and injury prevention are based upon assessment of risks, learning theory, epidemiological principles, and the health beliefs and practices of the patient.

2. Methods of health promotion, maintenance, and teaching are appropriate to the developmental level, learning needs, readiness and ability to learn, and culture of the patient.

STANDARD 5D. PRESCRIPTIVE AUTHORITY AND TREATMENT

The advanced practice vascular nurse prescribes both pharmacologic and nonpharmacologic interventions, procedures, and treatments in accordance with state and federal laws and regulations to treat illness and improve functional health or to provide preventive care to patients with vascular disease.

Measurement Criteria

1. Treatment interventions and procedures are prescribed according to the patient's healthcare needs and are based upon current knowledge, practice, and research.

2. Procedures are used and performed as needed in the delivery of comprehensive care.

3. Pharmacologic agents are prescribed based upon a knowledge of pharmacological and physiological principles.

4. Specific pharmacologic agents or treatments are prescribed based upon clinical indicators and upon the status and needs of the patient.

5. Intended effects and potential adverse effects of pharmacologic and non-pharmacologic treatments are monitored.

6. Appropriate information about intended effects, potential adverse effects, proposed prescription costs, and alternative treatments and procedures is provided to the patient.

STANDARD 5E. REFERRAL

The advanced practice vascular nurse identifies the need for additional care and makes referrals as needed.

Measurement Criteria

1. As the primary provider, the advanced practice vascular nurse facilitates continuity of care by implementing recommendations from referral sources.

2. The advanced practice vascular nurse refers directly to specific providers based upon patient needs with consideration of benefits and costs.

STANDARD 6. EVALUATION

The advanced practice vascular nurse evaluates the patient's progress in attaining expected outcomes.

Measurement Criteria

1. The accuracy of diagnoses and effectiveness of interventions is evaluated in relation to the patient's attainment of the expected outcomes.

2. The evaluation process is based on advanced knowledge, practice, and research, and results in revision or resolution of diagnoses, expected outcomes, and plan of care.

ADVANCED PRACTICE
STANDARDS OF PROFESSIONAL PERFORMANCE

STANDARD 1. QUALITY OF CARE

The advanced practice vascular nurse develops criteria for and evaluates the quality of care and effectiveness of advanced practice vascular nursing.

Measurement Criteria

The advanced practice vascular nurse:

1. Assumes, as the clinical expert, a leadership role in establishing and monitoring standards of practice to improve patient care.

2. Uses the results of quality-of-care analysis to initiate changes throughout the healthcare system as appropriate.

3. Participates in efforts to minimize costs and unnecessary duplication of testing or other diagnostic activities and to facilitate timely treatment of the vascular patient.

4. Reviews factors related to safety, satisfaction, effectiveness, and cost/benefit options with the patient, and other providers as appropriate.

5. Analyzes organizational systems for barriers and promotes enhancements that affect healthcare status of the vascular patient.

6. Bases their evaluation on current knowledge, practice, and research.

7. Seeks professional certification in the area of vascular nursing.

STANDARD 2. SELF-EVALUATION

The advanced practice vascular nurse continuously evaluates one's own vascular nursing practice in relation to professional practice standards and relevant statutes and regulations, and is accountable to the public and to the profession for providing competent clinical care.

Measurement Criteria

The advanced practice vascular nurse:

1. Has the inherent responsibility as a professional to evaluate one's own performance according to the standards of the profession and various regulatory bodies, and to take action to improve practice.

2. Seeks feedback regarding one's own practice and role performance from peers, professional colleagues, patients and others.

3. Self-evaluates practice based on patient outcomes.

STANDARD 3. EDUCATION

The advanced practice vascular nurse acquires and maintains current knowledge and skills in the specialty area of vascular nursing.

Measurement Criteria

The advanced practice vascular nurse:

1. Uses current healthcare research to expand clinical knowledge, enhance role performance, and increase knowledge of professional issues.

2. Seeks formal experiences or independent learning activities to maintain and develop clinical and professional skills and knowledge.

STANDARD 4. LEADERSHIP

The advanced practice vascular nurse serves as a leader and role model for the professional development of peers, colleagues, and others.

Measurement Criteria

The advanced practice vascular nurse:

1. Contributes to the professional development of others to improve patient care and to foster the profession's growth.

2. Brings creativity and innovation to nursing practice to improve delivery of care.

3. Participates in professional activities.

4. Works to influence policy-making bodies to improve patient care.

5. Fosters a learning environment when mentoring and preceptoring students.

STANDARD 5. ETHICS

The advanced practice vascular nurse integrates ethical principles and norms in all areas of practice.

Measurement Criteria

The advanced practice vascular nurse:

1. Maintains a therapeutic and professional relationship and discusses the delineation of roles and parameters of the relationship with the patient.

2. Informs the patient of potential risks, benefits, and outcomes of healthcare regimens.

3. Contributes to resolving the ethical dilemmas of individuals or systems.

STANDARD 6. INTERDISCIPLINARY PROCESS

The advanced practice vascular nurse promotes an interdisciplinary process in providing patient care.

Measurement Criteria

The advanced practice vascular nurse:

1. Works with other disciplines to enhance patient care; interdisciplinary activities may include education, consultation, management, technological development, or research opportunities.

2. Facilitates an interdisciplinary process with other members of the healthcare team.

STANDARD 7. RESEARCH

The advanced practice vascular nurse uses research findings to discover, examine, and evaluate knowledge, theories, and creative approaches to healthcare practices.

Measurement Criteria

The advanced practice vascular nurse:

1. Critically evaluates existing practice in light of current research findings.

2. Identifies research questions in practice.

3. Disseminates relevant research findings through practice, education, or consultation.

GLOSSARY

Assessment. A systematic, dynamic process by which the nurse, through interaction with the patient, significant others, and healthcare providers, collects and analyzes data about the patient. Data may include the following dimensions: physical, psychological, socio-cultural, spiritual, cognitive, functional abilities, developmental, economic, and life-style.

Certification. The process by which a professional organization validates, based on predetermined standards, an individual registered nurse's qualification, knowledge, and practice in a defined functional or clinical area of nursing.

Continuity of care. An interdisciplinary process that includes patients, families, and significant others in the development of a coordinated plan of care. This process facilitates the patient's transition between settings and healthcare providers, based on changing needs and available resources.

Diagnosis (diagnosing). (1) The naming of the disease, illness, or syndrome a patient has or is believed to have, using classifications from various healthcare fields. (2) A clinical judgment to determine the state of health, disease, illness, or injury. Diagnosis depends upon the advanced synthesis of information obtained during the interview, physical exam, or diagnostic test.

Differential diagnosis. The determination of which of two or more diseases with similar symptoms is most applicable, leaving only one disease to which all the symptoms point.

Environment. The atmosphere, milieu, or conditions in which an individual lives, works, or plays.

Evaluation. The process of determining both the patient's progress toward the attainment of expected outcomes and the effectiveness of nursing care by systematic appraisal and study.

Evidence-based practice. A process founded on the collection, interpretation, and integration of valid, important, and applicable patient-reported, clinician-observed, and research-derived evidence. The best available evidence, moderated by patient circumstances and preferences, is applied to improve the quality of clinical judgments.

Family. Family of origin or significant others as identified by the patient.

Healthcare providers. People with special expertise who provide healthcare services or assistance to patients. They may include nurses, pharmacists, physicians, psychologists, social workers, nutritionists/dietitians, and various other therapists.

Implementation. Activities such as teaching, monitoring, providing, counseling, delegating and coordinating.

Implementation outcome. The end result of a learning activity measured by written evaluation or change in practice.

Interdisciplinary. Reliant on the overlapping skills and knowledge of each team member and discipline, resulting in synergistic effects where outcomes are enhanced and more comprehensive than the simple aggregation of any team member's individual efforts.

Patient. Recipient of nursing care. The term *patient* rather than *client* is used in this document and may represent an individual (the focus is on the health state, problems, or needs of a single person), family or group (the focus is on the health state of the unit as a whole or the reciprocal effects of an individual's health state on the other members of the unit), or community (the focus is on the personal and environmental health and the health risks of population groups).

Plan. A comprehensive outline of the components that need to be addressed to attain expected outcomes.

Prescriptive authority. Those nurses who are credentialed as advanced practitioners and who follow statutes, rules, and regulations as determined by each individual state.

Quality of care. The degree to which health services for patients, families, groups, communities, or populations increase the likelihood of desired outcomes and are consistent with current professional knowledge.

Standard. Authoritative statement enunciated and promulgated by the profession, by which the quality of practice, service, or education can be judged.

Standards of care. Authoritative statements that describe a competent level of clinical nursing practice demonstrated through assessment, diagnosis, outcome identification, planning, implementation, and evaluation.

Standards of nursing practice. Authoritative statements that describe a level of care or performance common to the profession of nursing by which the quality of nursing practice can be judged and reassured.

Standards of professional performance. Authoritative statements that describe a competent level of behavior in the professional role, including activities related to quality of care, performance appraisal, education, collegiality, ethics, collaboration, research, and resource utilization.

REFERENCES

American Heart Association. (2004). *Heart disease and stroke statistics—2004 Update.* Dallas, TX: American Heart Association.

American Nurses Association. (1996). *Scope and standards of advanced practice registered nursing.* Washington, DC: American Nurses Publishing.

American Nurses Association. (1998). *Standards of clinical nursing practice, 2nd edition.* Washington, DC: American Nurses Publishing.

American Nurses Association. (2001). *Code of ethics for nurses with interpretive statements.* Washington, DC: American Nurses Publishing.

American Nurses Credentialing Center Commission on Certification. (2001). *Cardiac/Vascular nurse computer-based testing catalog.* Washington, DC: American Nurses Credentialing Center.

American Stroke Association and JCAHO Collaborate on JCAHO's Primary Stroke Center Certification Program. (2003). Available at www.jcaho.org.

de Araujo, T., Valencia, I., Federman, F., & Kirsner, R.S. (2003). Managing the patient with venous ulcers. *Annals of Internal Medicine,* 138 (4), 326–334.

Beckman, J., Creager, M., & Libby, P. (2003). Diabetes and atherosclerosis: Epidemiology, pathophysiology and management. *Journal of the American Medical Association,* 287 (7), 2570–2581.

Canto, J.G., & Iskandrian, A.E. (2003). Major risk factors for cardiovascular disease: Debunking the only 50% myth. *Journal of the American Medical Association,* 290 (7), 947–949.

Criqui, M.H., Langer, R.D., & Fronek, A. (1992). Mortality over a period of 10 years in patients with peripheral arterial disease. *New England Journal of Medicine,* 326, 381–386.

Gillum, R. F. (1995). Epidemiology of aortic aneurysm in the United States. *Journal of Clinical Epidemiology,* 48 (11), 1289–298.

Hackam, D.G., & Anand, S.S. (2003). Emerging risk factors for atherosclerotic vascular disease: A clinical review of evidence. *Journal of the American Medical Association,* 290 (7), 932–940.

Hiatt, R.F., & Cooke, J.P. (2001). Medical treatment of peripheral arterial disease and claudication. *New England Journal of Medicine,* 344, 1608–1621.

Makary, M.A. (2001). *Aortic stent grafts: Technology briefing for cardiovascular leaders. Cardiovascular Roundtable.* Washington, DC: The Advisory Board Company.

Mitchell, M.B., Rutherford, R.B., & Krupski, W.C. (1999). Infrarenal Aortic Aneurysms. In R.B. Rutherford, P. Gloviczki & J.L Cronenwett (Eds.), *Vascular surgery (5th ed.).* Philadelphia: Harcourt Brace & Company.

National Diabetes Information Clearinghouse. *Diabetes across the United States.* http://diabetes.niddk.nih.gov/populations/index.htm. Accessed on January 14, 2004.

Ouriel, K. (2001). Detection of peripheral arterial disease in primary care. *Journal of the American Medical Association,* 286 (11), 1380–1381.

Treat-Jacobson, D., & Walsh, M.E. (2003). Treating patients with peripheral arterial disease and claudication. *Journal of Vascular Nursing.* 21 (1), 5–14.

Verloes, A., Sakalihasan, A., & Limet, R. (1995). Aneurysms of the abdominal aorta: Familial and genetic aspects in three hundred and thirteen pedigrees. *Journal of Vascular Surgery,* 21, 646–655.

INDEX

A

Abdominal aortic aneurysm (AAA), 3–4
   See also Vascular disease
Activity, 6
   See also Vascular nursing:
     phenomena of concern
Advanced practice vascular nursing, 2, 8–9
   assessment, 27
   case management and
     coordination of care, 29
   consultation, 30
   diagnosis, 27
   education, 34
   ethics, 35
   evaluation, 32
   health promotion, health
     maintenance, and health
     teaching, 30
   implementation, 36
   interdisciplinary process, 36
   leadership, 35
   outcome identification, 28
   planning, 28
   prescriptive authority and
     treatment, 31
   quality of care, 33
   referral, 32
   research, 36
   self-evaluation, 34
   See also Generalist vascular
     nursing; Vascular nursing
Advocacy for patients and families, 10, 23
Age-appropriate care. *See* Cultural
   competence
Alternative therapies, 10

American Nurses Association (ANA), 11
American Nurses Credentialing
   Center, 9
Analysis. *See* Critical thinking,
   analysis, and synthesis
Assessment, 1, 2, 5
   in advanced practice, 8, 9
   defined, 37
   diagnosis and, 14, 27
   ethics and, 23
   evaluation and, 18
   health promotion and, 7
   implementation and, 17
   outcome identification and, 28
   planning and, 28
   standard of care, 13, 27

B

Boards on Certification (BOC), 9

C

Care recipient. *See* Patient
Care standards. *See* Standards of care
Case management and coordination
   of care
   planning and, 16
   standard of care, 29
Cerebrovascular disease. *See* Stroke
Certification and credentialing, 8, 9
   defined, 37
   quality of care and, 33
Chronic venous insufficiency, 4–5
   See also Vascular disease
Circulation, 5
   See also Vascular nursing:
     phenomena of concern
Client. *See* Patient
Clinical settings. *See* Practice settings

Documentation
    assessment and, 13
    diagnosis and, 14
    evaluation and, 18
    implementation and, 17
    outcome identification and, 15
    planning and, 16, 28

E
Economic issues. *See* Cost control
Education of vascular nurses
    collaboration and, 24
    collegiality and, 22
    curriculum, 8
    importance of, 9, 11
    implementation and, 17
    interdisciplinary process and, 36
    quality of care and, 19
    research and, 25, 36
    standard of professional
        performance, 21, 34
    See also Professional
        development
Education of patients and families
    abdominal aortic aneurysm
        (AAA) and, 4
    consultation and, 30
    diabetes and, 3
    ethics and, 23, 35
    health promotion and, 6–7, 30
    planning and, 16
    resource utilization and, 26
    trends, 11
    venous disease and, 5
    See also Family; Health
        promotion, health
        maintenance, and health
        teaching; Patient
Environment
    defined, 37
    vascular disease and, 5–6
    See also Practice environment

Ethics, 10
    codes, 9, 10, 23
    implementation and, 17
    research and, 25
    standard of professional
performance, 23, 35
    See also Laws, statutes, and
        regulations
Evaluation
    in advanced practice, 9
    assessment and, 7
    defined, 37
    outcome identification and, 28
    prescriptive authority and, 31
    quality of care and, 19, 33
    standard of care, 18, 32
Evidence-based practice
    consultation and, 30
    defined, 37
    education and, 34
    evaluation and, 32
    implementation and, 17, 29
    outcome identification and, 15, 28
    planning and, 16
    prescriptive authority and, 31
    quality of care and, 33
    See also Research

F
Family
    assessment and, 13
    collaboration and, 24
    defined, 37
    diagnosis and, 14
    ethics and, 10
    evaluation and, 18
    health promotion and, 6
    outcome identification and, 15
    quality of care and, 19
    as recipients of care, 1, 8
    resource utilization and, 26

Interventions, 2, 4, 7
   in advanced practice, 9
   assessment and, 27
   ethics and, 10, 23
   evaluation and, 18
   implementation and, 17, 29
   planning and, 16, 28
   prescriptive authority and, 31
   research and, 25

J
Journal of Vascular Nursing, 11

L
Laws, statutes, and regulations, 9
   ethics and, 23
   performance appraisal and, 20
   prescriptive authority and, 31
   resource utilization and, 26
   self-evaluation and, 34
   See also Ethics
Leadership
   advanced practice and, 8
   quality of care and, 33
   standard of professional
      performance, 35
Legal issues. *See* Laws, statutes, and
   regulations
Licensing. *See* Certification and
   credentialing
Lymphatic disease, 5
   See *also* Vascular disease

M
Maintaining function, 1, 7
Management of vascular disease, 3,
   7, 8, 9
   See also Vascular disease
Measurement criteria. *See* Criteria for
   standards

Mentoring
   collegiality and, 22
   leadership and, 35
Multidisciplinary healthcare. *See*
   Interdisciplinary healthcare

N
National Institutes of Health,
Non-atherosclerotic arterial disease, 4
   See also Vascular disease
Nursing care standards. *See*
   Standards of care
Nursing Organization Alliance, 11
Nursing standards. *See* Standards of
   care; Standards of professional
   performance
Nutrition, 6
   See also Vascular nursing:
      phenomena of concern

O
Outcome identification
   standard of care, 15, 28
   See also Outcomes
Outcomes
   in advanced practice, 9
   case management and, 29
   defined, 38
   diagnosis and, 14
   ethics and, 35
   evaluation and, 18, 32
   health promotion and, 7
   implementation and, 17
   planning and, 16, 28
   quality of care and, 19
   research and, 25
   resource utilization and, 26
   self-evaluation and, 34
   See also Outcome identification

resource utilization and, 26
standard of professional
  performance, 19, 33
Quality of life
  outcome identification and, 51
  planning and, 16
  quality of care and, 19

R

Recipient of care. *See* Patient
Referral
  collaboration and, 24
  planning and, 16
  resource utilization and, 26
  standard of care, 32
Regaining function, 1, 7
Regulatory issues. See Laws, statutes,
  and regulations
Research
  in advanced practice, 8, 9
  assessment and, 27
  collaboration and, 10, 24
  diagnosis and, 14
  education and, 34
  evaluation and, 18, 32
  future trends, 10
  implementation and, 17, 29
  interdisciplinary process and, 36
  planning and, 16, 28
  prescriptive authority and, 31
  quality of care and, 33
  standard of professional
    performance, 25, 36
  in vascular nursing, 1
  See also Evidence-based practice
Resource utilization, 11
  ethics and, 23
  standard of professional
    performance, 26
Response to illness, 6
  See also Vascular nursing:
    phenomena of concern

Rest, 6
  See also Vascular nursing:
    phenomena of concern
Risk assessment
  ethics and, 35
  health promotion and, 30
  outcome identification and, 28
  planning and, 16
  prescriptive authority and, 31
  quality of care and, 19
  resource utilization and, 26
Risk factors for vascular disease, 1, 2,
  7, 11
  diagnosis and, 14
  quality of care and, 19

S

Safety assurance, 10
  collegiality and, 22
  implementation and, 17
  quality of care and, 33
  resource utilization and, 26
Scientific findings. *See* Evidence-
  based practice; Research
Scope of practice, *vii*, 1–11
  advanced level, 8–9
  generalist level, 8
Self-care and self-management, 6, 11
  planning and, 16
  See also Vascular nursing:
    phenomena of concern
Self-evaluation
  standard of professional
    performance, 34
Sensation, 6
  See also Vascular nursing:
    phenomena of concern
Settings. *See* Practice settings
Significant others. *See* Family
Skin integrity, 6
  See also Vascular nursing:
    phenomena of concern

Sleep, 6
    See also Vascular nursing:
        phenomena of concern
Smoking cessation, 11
Society for Vascular Nursing (SVN),
    vii, 11
Standard (defined), 38
Standards of care, *viii*, 9, 13–18,
    27–32
    assessment, 13, 27
    case management and
        coordination of care, 29
    consultation, 30
    defined, 38
    diagnosis, 14, 27
    evaluation, 18, 32
    health promotion, health
        maintenance, and health
        teaching, 30
    implementation, 17, 29–32
    outcome identification, 15, 28
    planning, 16, 28
    prescriptive authority and
        treatment, 31
    referral, 32
Standards of practice, *viii*
    defined, 38
    See also Standards of care
Standards of professional
    performance, *viii*, 19–26, 33–36
    collaboration, 24
    collegiality, 22
    defined, 38
    education, 21, 34
    ethics, 23, 35
    interdisciplinary process, 36
    leadership, 35
    performance appraisal, 20
    quality of care, 19, 33
    research, 25, 36
    resource utilization, 26
    self-evaluation, 34

Statistics of vascular disease, 2, 3, 4, 5
Stroke, 4
    See also Vascular disease
Synthesis. *See* Critical thinking,
    analysis, and synthesis

T
Teaching. *See* Education; Health
    promotion, health maintenance,
    and health teaching
Teams and teamwork. *See*
    Interdisciplinary healthcare
Trends in vascular nursing, 10–11

V
Vascular disease, 1–5
    abdominal aortic aneurysm
        (AAA), 3–4
    arterial disease, 1–4
    chronic venous insufficiency
        (CVI), 4–5
    defined, 1
    diabetes mellitus and, 2–3
    lymphatic disease, 5
    management of, 3, 7
    nonatherosclerotic arterial
        disease, 4
    peripheral arterial disease (PAD),
        1–2
    risk factors, 1, 2, 7
    statistics, 2, 3, 4, 5
    venous disease, 4–5
Vascular Disease Foundation, 11
Vascular nursing, *vii*
    advanced practice, 8–9
    certification, 9
    characteristics, 5–6
    defined, 1
    ethics, 10
    generalist practice, 8
    health promotion and, 6–7
    phenomena of concern, 5–6

W

ANA NURSING STANDARDS PACKAGE

The set—totaling over 1,000 pages—contains **the newly revised keystone publication of the set,** *Nursing: Scope and Standards of Practice,* **plus one each of the current volume for the 22 nursing specialty areas** listed below. Each volume delineates and discusses the scope, status, and prospects of that specialized practice along with its generalist competencies, any advanced practice competencies, and the evidence-based standards with measurement criteria for practice and professional performance.

Pub# PKG   *List $330/Member $260*

The ANA Standards Package contains:

NURSING: SCOPE AND STANDARDS OF PRACTICE, 2004/126 pp. (*NEW EDITION*)
   Provides the standards for clinical, non-clinical, and advanced practice; includes the 1973, 1981, 1991, and 1997 editions.
#04SSNP   **List $19.95/Member $16.95**

... plus 22 additional scope and standards of specialty practice*, all affordably priced at List $16.95/Member $13.45:
The latest additions to the set...

Nurse Administrators, 2004 (*NEW EDITION*)	#03SSNA	**Nursing Professional Development**, 2000	#NPD20
Addictions Nursing, 2004 (*NEW EDITION*)	#04SSAN	**Palliative & Hospice Nursing**, 2002	#HPN22
Neonatal Nursing, 2004 (*FIRST EDITION*)	#04SSNN	**Parish Nursing**, 1998	#9806ST
Vascular Nursing, 2004 (*FIRST EDITION*)	#04SSVN	**Pediatric Nursing**, 2003 (*NEW EDITION*)	#PNP23
... join		**Pediatric Oncology Nursing**, 2000	#PONP20
College Health Nursing, 1997	# ST1	**Psychiatric–Mental Health Nursing**, 2000	#PMH20
Correctional Facilities Nursing, 1995	#NP104	**Public Health Nursing**, 1999	#910PH
Developmental Disabilities		**School Nursing**, 2001	#SHNP21
and/or Mental Retardation, 1998	#9802ST		
Diabetes Nursing, 2nd Edition, 2003	#DNP23		
Forensic Nursing, 1997	#ST4		
Genetics Clinical Nursing, 1998	#9807ST		
Gerontological Nursing, 2nd Edition, 2001	#GNP21		
Home Health Nursing, 1999	#9905HH		
Neuroscience Nursing, 2002	#NNS22		
Nursing Informatics, 2001	#NIP21		

ANA STANDARDS STANDING ORDER PLAN

Great plan for university, hospital, and medical center libraries! Get the newest Standards as soon as they are published. We'll send the book along with an invoice. Plus, you'll save 10% off list price.
(ANA members receive an additional 20% savings.)
For details, or to enroll, call (800) 637-0323.

(* Titles may be ordered separately.)

ORDER FORM

Title	Price	Qty	Total
Nursing Standards Package #PKG			
	Shipping & Handling		
TOTAL			.

Shipping and Handling		
	U.S.	Outside U.S.
Up to $25	$4	$8
25.01–$50	$6	$12
$50.01–$100	$8	$16
$100.01–$200	$14	$24
$200.01–$300	$12	$32
$300.01^{+}	7% of total	15% of total

Shipping: 7–10 days for domestic deliveries. 7–30 business days for international deliveries. Items cannot be delivered to a P.O. box. All orders must include shipping and handling charges.

Payment: (payment in U.S. dollars required)
[ ] Check enclosed (made payable to *American Nurses Association*)
Charge my [ ] VISA   [ ] MasterCard

Card # _____ Exp Date _____

Signature _____

Phone # _____ CMA# _____ **

** *Your CMA I.D. number must be provided to receive member discount.*
   20% discount off list price on orders of 20+ copies of the same title.

Ship to:
Name _____

Organization _____

Address _____

City/State/Zip _____

Phone # _____ Fax # _____

HOW TO ORDER

Online: WWW.NURSESBOOKS.ORG **Phone**: 800/637-0323   **Fax**: 770/280-4141 **Mail**: nursesbooks.org, P.O. Box 931895, Atlanta, GA 31193-1895